SURVIVING COVID-19

HOW DID I GET HERE?

JAMEEL MCKANSTRY

13TH & JOAN

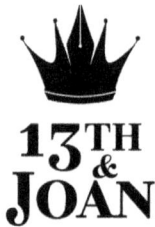

For permission requests, write to the publisher, addressed "Attention: Permissions Coordinator," 205 N. Michigan Avenue, Suite #810, Chicago, IL 60601. 13th & Joan books may be purchased for educational, business or sales promotional use. For information, please email the Sales Department at sales@13thandjoan.com.

Printed in the U. S. A.

First Printing, May 2022.

Library of Congress Cataloging-in-Publication Data has been applied for.

ISBN: 978-1-953156-73-0

To Summer, Amier, and Caden

"Written with humor and stark honesty, this book is a testament to the power of human connection…"

Jeff MacCulloch

"…I loved the humanistic approach to capture a man in the throes of a pandemic during a time where we are forced into such "un-human" conditions…"

Ta'Qoyia "Taco" Thomas

"..I, too, felt a whole range of emotions while reading it - I laughed, I cried a few tears, but most of all I was touched by your honesty, sincerity, and your love and appreciation for your life and all those who are in it…"

Greg Kilpatrick

"When I began this book, I was sure that I had no desire to read about Covid-19. It quickly proved me wrong! Reading about Jameel's experience is like speaking to a friend–it is an emotionally intelligent account of what it was like to have the scariest virus around in the midst of the worst part of the pandemic, and it left me feeling almost uplifted…"

Meghan Nickerson

Foreword

ERHAPS ONE OF THE MOST COMPLEX QUESTIONS THAT stump theologians and the everyday person alike is: *"Why do bad things happen to good people?"* Much of this complexity is rooted in a general perception that God is "always good" and that if one prays, fasts, and follows God that there is a protection from destruction. However, people who follow God are required to possess a greater level of maturity when approaching bad and or/traumatic life events. Perhaps one of the most mature scriptures in the Bible is found in Romans 8:28. It reads: *"For we know all things work together for the good of them who love the Lord and have been called unto his purpose which is in Christ Jesus."* This scripture is an uncanny trust that the sum total of one's life events at some point will make sense and produce "a particular good". The key component to this scripture in my mind is found in this part: *"for the good of them who love the Lord."* One must love God in order to trust that the live events that unfold in one's life will produce some good from the bad. When one is loved God, it is having an understanding that "for the good" means accepting that what happens to us produces internal growth and elevated perspective.

Jameel McKanstry is considered a part of *"those who love God."* While I am never certain about God's decisions, I have learned God knows who can be entrusted to endure life circumstances and give glory to God in and out of the circumstance. Such perspective turns the question from "Why Jameel?" to "Why not Jameel?" In this story, the very gift- his voice- that made him exceptional - was the very area under attack. The inability to breathe. His lungs, at the risk of collapse.

Jameel has numerous characteristics that make his story worthy of highlighting to the world. Perhaps his most cherished characteristic is his rich and versatile human instrument, which I heard about before meeting him in person during his freshman year at Florida State University. In fact, his voice preceded him during that time on the campus of Florida State University. Jameel's voice feels rooted like a good Baptist service on a Sunday morning and filled with warmth and the feeling that "he is living an honest life". Jameel comes from a place where how you live your life overrides the gift. When we finally met, I made him perform a musical *"run"* on the spot. Slightly taken aback, he rose to the occasion and that moment marked the beginning of a profound relationship to the time of this book. Just when I thought our connection could not get any better, he worked hard and sacrificed to become a member of my beloved fraternity, Alpha Phi Alpha Fraternity, Incorporated.

Undeniably our most significant bond that I also knew almost immediately was his deep connection to the Black church. He comes from a place where you went to church at least three days a week before Sunday because Choir rehearsal had to happen. A place where you'd be cut like a blade by a shady aunt or church mother. They would give you a compliment just to give you a critique. He comes from the smell of chicken fried to perfection and the taste of sweet tea- the kind that contributes to diabetes down the line if not careful. The place where the auntie's sole purpose in life is to make a macaroni cheese that makes everyone jealous at family gatherings, especially Thanksgiving. Hymns. Deacons and deaconesses. The lived experience of witnessing the Holy Ghost move in and out of during and/or after a hymn that had the mothers reflect on how God had kept them "down through the years". From the South, and more specifically, the smaller cities and towns produces in my mind the most balanced people. People who are rooted and relentless and resourceful. Gritty and guided. Purposeful and polite and so many other attributes. This was and still is our shared language and experience. I remember being able to see a version of myself when I met him as a freshman.

I was not surprised when New York City called his name to settle even at the time of this book. I believe wholeheartedly that at some point, whether one wants to live here or not, NYC should call your name to exercise your talents. Like a proud big brother, I have been incredibly proud of his perseverance to complete a master's program at a reputable NYC-based institution; the gift to educate young and eager minds in the upper West Side of Manhattan, and most importantly raise a family in the most boisterous and decorated city in the world.

I, too, remember when I got the phone call about Jameel's admittance into the hospital for COVID in the wake of the global pandemic. I was only able to pray that God's will would be to grant him the chance to survive. In a later conversation with Jameel, I reminded him that grace kept him here. Nothing else explains why his life was spared and hundreds of thousands of others lost their lives. The truth is, sometimes we can pray for the healing of a loved one and still lose them. It's about God's sovereignty on whether we succumb to or survive life threatening situations.

I cannot say with confidence why God granted grace for Jameel to live. What I do know is God knows all things and knew Jameel would turn his battle with COVID-19 into a testimony with the goal of inspiring and empowering others to trust God at all times, even when things aren't favorable. To be clear, each of us has the prerogative to shield or share our stories. I am grateful Jameel chose the latter. Perhaps it is one reason why he is still here with us today. In many ways, remaining in silos prevents us from experiencing the value of connection. Jameel chose to share instead of shield what happened to him along with millions of others across the world. As I close my thoughts, I strongly encourage each of us to tap into the power of sharing our stories. Let us share our stories because of the power of highlighting possibilities when others cannot detect it in their own journey at times.

I often say to people as I preach and counsel them at various stages of life how important it is to retreat to a "crew" instead of a "cave" when tumultuous life moments happen. There will be moments in life where we will not have the capacity to handle what life presents to us and give out of steam. This is why a "crew" and partnership is needed to press toward the miracle we need for healing. The power of family and community was apparent as he walked us through the most scary moment of his life. I have the privilege of knowing his wife Summer, another countless member of Black Girl Magic, his ultra talented boys, and the scores of loyal and lifetime fraternity brothers. The flashbacks of seeing faces you love and love you back usually provide that extra kick - that extra push to keep living. Let the record reflect that Jameel McKanstry has a metropolis of beautiful people who respect, adore and love him endlessly and others will after hearing his story.

I am grateful that this book is one that celebrates a beloved father, son, friend, uncle, educator and numerous other meaningful roles who conquered COVID-19. We must never forget, however, the millions of lives that succumbed to this virus, and therefore let's constantly pray and send warm thoughts and positive energy for families and friends who will forever mourn their precious lives since 2020 and at the time of this book.

Donald C. Garner, PhD

Emergency

"911, WHAT'S YOUR EMERGENCY?"

"I have had symptoms of COVID 19 for almost two weeks, and now I'm having a hard time breathing."

"Okay, sir, I need some information."

I gave the 911 operator my address, but I could tell my memory was extremely fuzzy. I had been in quarantine in my bedroom for two weeks. I was having several symptoms of COVID 19: chills, fever, extreme fatigue, oh, and mucus. Lots of mucus. Though my memory was fading, I was able to fight through it and give the 911 operator the information they needed to send help. I never called 911 before this day. Well...there were those times I called when I was a child, but this time, I needed help. Emergency response help. As I got dressed, I heard my wife, Summer, call upstairs in a loud voice, "Babe, did you call 911? They're here." I tried to hurry as best I could and went downstairs to hug her, our two boys, and my mother-in-law. The expressions on their faces varied. My wife and mother-in-law looked gravely concerned, while my six-year-old, Amier, looked confused. Caden, who was nine months at the time, looked like any baby, hungry.

I was in danger of losing my life. What would my wife do without me? My children? My mom? My brothers? So much was in the balance as I slowly walked out of the house. I remember like it was yesterday. I was wearing gray camouflage pants, a gray hoodie, and black sneakers with no socks because I knew I would get those infamous hospital socks-*you know*, the ones with the grippers? Yep, those. As I walked out of our home, I could feel the cold chill from the air on my ankles, and my thoughts began to race. *Maybe I should have grabbed socks. How long am I gonna be in the hospital? Did I remember to pay my phone bill? Ugh.* -Mr. McKanstry? The EMT interrupted, "What is your date of birth." It took me a second, but I was able to give her my date of birth as I laid down on the stretcher and was strapped in. And just like that, I was on my way to the hospital. I watched as we drove away, and my home became smaller and smaller. I couldn't help thinking to myself, *how did I get here?* Let's go back to a few weeks prior. Here's where it all started.

Among the many things that I am, I'm also a musician. I started playing piano at the age of four. Growing up in Tuscaloosa,AL., I have fond memories of playing the piano in the house with my friends, playing church, and all that. I grew up in a devout Christian home, and in addition to my mom's four other jobs, she played piano for the church. I loved going to choir rehearsals, and I loved to hear the saints at my home church, New Prospect Missionary Baptist Church, sing songs like "I Love the Lord, He Heard My Cry" and "I Know I Been Changed." This experience molded me and shaped me into the musician I am today. Fast forward almost thirty years, and I'm still playing and singing in church.

In March of 2020, the world was in an uproar. New York City Schools, a public school system with 1800 public schools, shut down. As a teacher, I felt prepared-as prepared as we could be. My school did an excellent job preparing staff and students for an imminent lockdown that would change schools and life for the foreseeable future. At this point, I had been teaching music for ten years and even started the music program at Lafayette Academy, an amazing middle school community on the Upper West Side of Manhattan. At the time of the shutdown, we were in the middle of rehearsals for "High School Musical, Jr." The previous school year, our students successfully put on "Lion King, Jr." It was such a powerful moment for our school and the community. At the last show of "Lion King, Jr.," we announced we'd be putting up High School Musical, Jr. The room roared with excitement. It was electrifying. If I had ever had any doubts, I knew then I was in the right place at just the right time. So as you could imagine, the students, who had spent their time learning the lines, music, and choreography for a show that was no longer going to happen, were crushed. I was crushed. Truthfully, I was never able to really process the loss of this show. There was just so much going on. Our world had instantly changed, and we didn't know if it would ever be the same.

Of course, along with schools being shut down, gatherings of any kind were almost nonexistent. Like most industries and organizations, the church also had to pivot during this time. My church went to a virtual model where a small group would come in and film the service, then broadcast on Facebook Live for the rest of the congregation. Several churches adopted this same model. So somewhere between my weekly grocery store run and my weekly church attendance, I got COVID 19. One of the terrible things about this sickness is that you can't pinpoint exactly when it was contracted, at least not to my knowledge. However, I do remember my last time out of the house before I started feeling sick. That was on Resurrection Sunday. The Sunday in Christian faith that commemorates Jesus, the Son of God, being raised from the dead, having been crucified three days prior. I had resolved that this would be my last Sunday for a while because COVID 19 cases were really starting to pick up, and New York City was the epicenter of the world. Every day my mom and brothers called me to make sure I was being safe-masking up, sanitizing, and social distancing. Honestly, I was. I was always wearing my mask. At this time, I was even wearing gloves everywhere and just taking them off to play the organ. Regardless of where I got it from, the fact is I got it, and it would manifest itself within the next few days. The week prior to Resurrection Sunday, our car, a 2014 Jeep Grand Cherokee, stopped while I was getting groceries. Picture this, after I loaded up the groceries in the car, I go to push the button to start the car, and it won't start. This was not the first time this had happened. So, I had to get a car service to bring me home and have my wife bring me back to be there when it was towed to the dealership. About a week later, on April 15, I went to pick up our car from the dealership. All of a sudden, while driving, I felt slightly tired. I struggled all the way home, went upstairs to bed, and fell asleep around four in the afternoon. I didn't wake up until the following day. I told my wife I wasn't feeling well, and we decided that I would start quarantining just to be on the safe side.

I remember being totally down for about two days. I was extremely fatigued and hardly ate anything-this isn't normal at all. I am a big guy. At this time, I was 5'11" and about 385 lbs. After those days passed, I was okay but was still quarantining. "*Babe*" said Summer in a low groan, from the open space next to our bedroom, "*I need you to take Caden to Ma. I am feeling so bad.*" These types of things are not normal for our family. We are not a sickly group of people. Furthermore, I'm a Southerner who believes strongly in home remedies so if anyone is sick, it doesn't usually last. I'll whip up some concoction usually with ginger or some other down home remedy and usually it does the trick. I'll tell you more about that later. Anyway, back to the story. Since Summer wasn't feeling well, I put my mask on, grabbed little Caden, our little light skinned bundle of joy, and took him downstairs to be with my Mother-in-Law, Roberta (Ma). "Lord ham mercy," said Ma. My mother-in-law often goes to a Southern accent when things are going awry. She's a born and bred New-Yorker who's beyond sweet, but like we always say, "don't let the cane fool ya." G-ma will rip you a new one if you take her there. "I just don't know what we gon' do," she said as she rocked Caden back to sleep. "Both of you are down?"While shaking my head, I said, "Well, Amier will have to be on his own and take care of himself."

Ma laughed while nodding, "Yep!" We both shared a laugh, which then turned to looks of concern as if we both knew this setup was not going to last long. I was still not feeling the best but had to struggle to make sure Ma had everything she needed for the baby. Formula…bottles… sippy cup…I tend to say things out loud, so I don't forget anything. She already had the diaper caddy next to her, and it had extra clothes, so this should be good enough.

Next, I went back to the kitchen to make sure Amier had access to a bowl for cereal and pulled it down from the top of the refrigerator. I also made sure he had access to some fruit, sandwich meat, and frozen pizzas. For three days, Ma took care of the boys for us. This was challenging because at the time, she was not able to move as well. But like mothers do, they make it happen no matter what. **Sidenote**: we are not worthy of Black women. The strength they have to exude on a daily basis is unparalleled.

A few days later, I was in my room (quarantining, of course), and my phone rang. It's Summer. *Babe, Ma just called me and said that she's not feeling well.* Okay, so at this point, we're out of options. So I hesitantly asked, "Well, how are you feeling?" She paused for a moment and said, *"Well I'm actually feeling much better,"* in an assuring tone. Something to note about my wife and best friend: she is an extreme realist, so if there had been anything wrong with her in the slightest way, she would have let me know. But she didn't. She was literally back to herself and able to take care of all of us. I told you, we are not worthy of women. I thank God every day for the special women he has placed in my life.

Over the course of the next few days, my symptoms took a turn for the worst. Headaches, fever, chills, fatigue, and no appetite filled my mornings, afternoons, and nights. I took all kinds of over-the-counter medication, but I could find no relief at all. I had even leaned on some of my remedies. I put a vapor-rub on my feet one night. Not really sure if it did anything. Another night, I put potatoes in my socks to try and draw the sickness out. I knew I was really sick because the potato slices were really dark. But I still wasn't getting better. At this point, I was starting to get nervous. Every day I watched as Gov. Andrew Cuomo gave updates on the numbers. They were spiking. The deaths were spiking. The next few days were a blur as I slept for most of them. But nothing could prepare me for what was next.

APRIL 23
Hallucinations, Alternate reality

S INCE THE START OF THE PANDEMIC, OUR STAFF HAD TO meet virtually every morning. We'd check-in and get any pertinent updates needed for remote learning. Even though I was quarantining, I still attended my morning meetings. However, today, April 23, 2020, this meeting was in a different environment. I have never told anyone about this. This meeting was being held underwater. I vividly remember laying on my bed and attending this meeting that was like an aquatic game of sorts with all types of fish. Each of my colleagues and I had a turn to play this underwater game and catch as many fish as we could. At the end of the meeting, I remember thinking, *"that was fun."*

Even more bizarre, I remember preparing our home for the underground aliens every day. They had invited me to join their team, and I was helping them with various tasks. If you're laughing, it's okay. I had to come to grips with the fact that I was in another place mentally. Truthfully, I was not prepared to be alone. Although some things were a bit hazy during this time, these memories are crystal clear. After diagnosing myself with COVID 19, I wanted to get the opinion of a medical professional so I had two virtual visits with two different doctors who gave me a few different prescriptions. Thank God for Summer, who went and got my meds. One of these medications was an antibiotic that made my stool loose. On this particular night, April 23, I remember listening to gospel music on my television. This song by The Clark Sisters, a world-renowned Gospel Group, was on. It had to be a little after midnight. In my dream, I was playing the piano for this legendary group and singing too. By the time I opened my eyes, I was standing up in my room, and while singing one of those high notes, I felt my bowels moving. How embarrassing!! Our bathroom was downstairs, and there was no way I could make it, so on the floor it went. Yuck! Thankfully I wasn't eating much, so it was pretty much a clear liquid. TMI … I know, but I want to tell you the truth, the whole truth. I used some baby wipes and sanitizer to clean myself up and went back to bed.

The next morning, I woke up to a knock on the door. "Come in," I said. Of course it was Summer coming in to check on me. She's about 5'7" and average weight. She leaned over, placed her hand on my head and said, "Babe, you're not doing any better. Maybe you should call and go to the hospital." Initially, I brushed it off like men tend to do. But my gut has always nudged me to listen to Summer.

She's special-gifted even. When I don't listen to her, things go poorly. I guess I've learned that over the last nearly fifteen years of knowing her. However, I was too prideful to tell her that I agree with her, so I kept my thoughts to myself. But trust me, my wheels were turning.

Elmhurst Hospital Day 1

O N April 24, 2020, around four in the afternoon, I was rushed into Elmhurst Hospital in Queens, NY. Just a few weeks earlier, this hospital was on Good Morning America as being the hospital with the most COVID 19 cases in the area. As they rushed me in, they took me to an area designated for COVID 19 patients. The room had beige floors and blinding fluorescent lights.

"All right, Mr. McKanstry, can you move yourself onto the bed?"

I hesitated for just a second, but I felt comfortable doing what the EMT requested. I told them I was cold, so the EMT gave me a bright green blanket. Immediately, I was enclosed in a material reminiscent of plastic Saran wrap. It was about three feet above my head. From there, everything kicked into high gear. Within what seemed like seconds, this team of doctors and nurses checked my vitals, took an x-ray, collected blood, and gave me an IV. There had to have been about ten of them. Everyone was so kind and attentive.

"Mr. McKanstry," one doctor said, "we're going to take good care of you." This eased some of my doubts, but to be honest, the heat from being surrounded in plastic like a holiday turkey had me feeling really uncomfortable. Even though the team of doctors seemed like they were moving at warp speed, this process still took more than two hours before I was in a room. As we left the chaos and entered the elevator, silence fell all around me.

It was close to seven in the evening. I had finally made it to my room. I video called my wife to let her see me. I could see a small version of myself. My beard was thick, black, and beat up. My usually bright eyes were sad and droopy. My face glistened from my rising body temperature. Summer was distraught. They put a BiPAP machine on my face to pump air into my body as I was not able to take in enough oxygen on my own-I was in respiratory distress, dehydrated, and extremely deficient in calcium and vitamin D. *"Babe, I'm so sorry. You look like you're going through a lot,"* she nearly cried. I answered her in a muffled tone, *"I'm okay babe. I feel pretty good."* This wasn't my first time in the hospital, but it was different. Because of the nature of this disease, my wife and best friend, who was always by my side, could not come to see me, and I had to be here alone. I told my wife that I was tired and would call her in the morning. We blew our kisses and said goodnight. I could hardly get comfortable with what felt like 30-45 mph winds blowing through me. So I closed my eyes. Suddenly I heard, *"Ohhhh. Get me out of here."* It was a moan from my roommate, a middle-aged man who was super slim. He had been in the hospital for a number of days, and the doctors had told him he was going home. This was obviously not happening tonight as the time was about eight. I had dealt with some interesting roommates in past hospital visits. Like this one time, an elderly gentleman was convinced that I was his wife and that I had all of his belongings; That I could deal with, but this…this was different. Every hour, my current roommate would call out for the nurse because he wanted to go home. Eventually, I tuned him out and went to sleep. Within what felt like minutes, I was awakened. *"Mr. McKanstry, we need to do another x-ray,"* the x-ray technician said. He put the ice cold machine on my chest and took the needed pictures. *"Mr. McKanstry, I'm your nurse. I need to check your vitals."* I let out a sigh of frustration muffled by the incessant noise from the BiPAP machine. "Your vitals are looking good," the nurse said as she took off the cuff for my blood pressure. She left quietly. I struggled to get comfortable. I had the compression devices squeezing my legs, an IV drip in my left arm, and yes, the BiPAP.

Let's face it, getting comfortable was not a thing tonight. *"Mr. McKanstry?"* As I was just about to close my eyes. "I'm Dr. Ritu. I've been reviewing your images. Your lungs are damaged. They look like shattered crystals. But don't lose hope. There's always hope." I'm only thirty-two years old. There's no way that I could be reaching the end of my life, could I? Many thoughts started to fill my head, but the scripture, Psalm 61:2, came to mind. "When my heart is overwhelmed, lead me to that rock that is higher than I." That night I prayed a simple prayer. *Dear Lord, I thank You for keeping me. Watch over me and protect me. I thank you for my healing. In Jesus' Name, Amen.* Shortly after that, I went to sleep.

The next morning, I was awakened by the nurses collecting blood, giving me my meds, and taking my vitals. Generally, every day, I'm thankful to be alive. However, while being hospitalized with a life-threatening disease that was killing thousands upon thousands, each new day was a big deal. Today was Saturday, and Saturdays are my favorite day of the week. We affectionately call it "family day." This Saturday was like no other. I was being poked and prodded, only to be then pumped with fluid, antibiotics, and medications. Not to mention, every day I received a shot in my thigh to prevent blood clots. It may sound like I'm complaining, but I assure you, I am so thankful for every measure the hospital staff took to save my life.

I grabbed my phone to check the time. It was six in the morning. I was wide awake, and there was no turning back at this point. So, I turned on the television. I love to cook, so I watch a lot of cooking shows. I'm pretty sure Diners Drive-Ins, and Dives was on, and the food was looking good. Within what felt like minutes, there was a knock on the door. It was time for breakfast; A banana, oatmeal, hot tea, and apple juice. At this point, I wasn't really convinced that I needed the BiPAP machine. After all, the day before, I was at home breathing moderately well. When I took off the BiPAP machine, there was no doubt. I wasn't gasping for air, but I felt like I needed to eat quickly so I could get the machine back on. As soon as I was done eating, that's just what I did. I was starting to feel light-headed as the Personal Care Assistant came in to help me put back on my BiPAP mask. My roommate left around ten this day, so it was a welcomed change to have the room to myself. Ahhh.

In undergrad, I joined the Infamous Iota Delta Chapter of Alpha Phi Alpha Fraternity, Inc., housed at Florida State University. I pledged with thirteen other guys, and they are forever my line brothers. While in undergrad, we were sure to make all plans for advancement in the university together. We worked hard to make those plans, whether that meant vying for positions in the Senate, Black Student Union, or even Alpha Phi Alpha on a state or regional level. I recall one of our meetings where I shared a scripture: 1 Corinthians 12. This chapter is about being one body with many parts. Each part of the body has its own function. So, it is with organizations. So, it is in business. The key is having all the right parts in place so they can function autonomously and in excellence. Those principles I spoke with them about nearly fourteen years ago still hold true today. Since we still think of ourselves as one, we try not to leave each other out of big life events. Most of them were able to come to our wedding. I have even attended a couple of weddings. I messaged them the day I went to the hospital.

It was awesome to read their well wishes in our group chat. Here are a few of my favorite:

> *I love you Huggie. I'm absolutely speechless right now. Fight my brother. Our God is greater than COVID.*
>
> *Just prayed and will continue to pray for you and your family. Fight like hell.*
>
> *Sorry to see this Huggie Bear. Prayers up for you and your family.*
>
> *You've got this Brother. We're here for you. We love you.*

Today, my line brother, Marvin, organized a line video call. I was reluctant to join. Thoughts immediately started to fill my head. *Did I really want them to see me like this? What would they think? What would they say?* I reluctantly pressed the link to join. Immediately I was met with familiar faces who were concerned and happy to see me. We went in line order onc through fourteen. We were all there. We updated each other on life experiences. When it was my turn, I shared with them how grateful I was to still have a steady income in the midst of a global pandemic. I told them that my family has not wanted for anything during this time, and for that, I was and still am eternally grateful. After everyone had finished sharing, a couple of laughs were shared, then we said our goodbyes. *That was awesome,* I thought to myself. Then my phone died. *Not a problem, I'll just get the charger out of my bag.* Then I remembered, I don't have a charger. Ugh. Now, if you are a millennial or know a millennial-yes, we millennials are in our thirties now-it is a sincere trepidation that comes over us when we're out with a dead phone. Immediately, I press the button to call the nurse. By now, they know they can't understand me through the speaker. A few minutes later, my PCA came in, and I asked her if she or anyone had an iPhone charger I could use. I'll check. I thanked her, asked for some more ice, and off she went. That night, I wasn't able to check social media and escape my situation. It was just me and basic cable. I turned to BET. They were doing a marathon of Tyler Perry movies. Madea's Family Reunion was playing. Johnny Gill was singing "You for Me." I sang this song as Summer walked down the aisle on our wedding day. Tears started to well up in my eyes, remembering how beautiful our wedding day was.

Picture this, Saturday, July 28, 2012. It was a pretty hot day in Tallahassee, FL. The time was four in the afternoon. It rained earlier that day, but thankfully it was just a passing, light storm. I was really nervous not only because my life was about to change forever, but I was pretty sure I lost my voice by drinking too much with my line brothers during my bachelor experience. I call it an experience because it was so much more than a party. Here I was in our church at the time, New Mount Zion. Throat scratchy, a little tired, but I was dressed and waiting for the day to begin. The thoughts began to race. *How will I know this will work out? How do you keep loving someone for years? Am I ready to be someone's husband?* All of those fears subsided when I saw those doors open to reveal my bride, Summer. She was a vision of perfection. Her hair was pulled into a bun, accented with pearls. Her skin was as golden as the sun at sunset. Her dress was stunning. Sparkly and pearly at the top and an elegant poof gently expanding to the floor. I was in awe of her beauty. I almost forgot I was supposed to sing. My hand was shaking as I started to sing. "It seems like forever..." As I continued to sing, I had to close my eyes to keep from crying. This was the moment that would be cemented in my mind for the rest of my life. The day we decided that we would tackle any obstacle never again alone-but together.

As I continued listening to Johnny Gill sing this song, the tears started to flow. I shed tears because I wasn't able to be there for my family. I shed tears because I was alone. I went to sleep and woke up in the middle of the night. It had to be around 1:00am. My throat was dry. My lips were chapped. Gusting air had been blowing through me for two days. I had learned how to take the mask off by myself by this point, so I did. I was just about to pour myself some water when all of a sudden I heard, *BEEEEP! BEEEEEEEEP!* The loudest beeps I had ever heard. It was the BiPAP machine. I guess patients aren't supposed to take off the mask without permission. I took a couple sips of water and was attempting to put the mask on when in came the night nurse. "Mr. McKanstry is everything okay?" I was embarrassed. I gently nodded, trying to pretend I had the mask on the whole time. "Now

Mr. McKanstry, we're gonna need you to keep your mask on.
We heard the machine beeping." I nodded again. I was even
more embarrassed, but I went back to sleep.

SUNDAY, APRIL 26
Elmhurst Hospital Day 3

"**M**R. *MCKANSTRY*," A MIDDLE-AGED WOMAN WITH beautiful brown skin and gray hair entered. "I am Mary, and I'm the Nurse Practitioner." I could tell by the way she spoke that she was not from New York. She had a southern accent that was pleasing and familiar to my ears. "Every day, I want you to pray. You've got to thank the Lord for another day. I want you to sit on the side of the bed. Take you some deep breaths. I mean, deep breaths and get up. Every day!! Walk around the room. Walk to the bathroom. Walk to the trash can. Get up out that bed. That bed will hold you and won't let you go. But you gotta get up and get outta here!"

Today was Sunday, and usually, I got to church on Sunday to hear a sermon from my Pastor. But Ms. Mary had given me a sermon before I could even get breakfast. So it was time for me to do what she said. I sat up, gave thanks for the day, and took some deep breaths. Being a classically trained singer, I was no stranger to taking deep breaths. *Inhale*...My deep breaths were interrupted by coughing. I could feel my lungs struggling to take in the amount of air that I was used to taking in. I teach my voice students to inhale up to four times so they can understand the true capacity of their lungs and stretch those muscles. But here I was, not even able to take a full breath without coughing.

Later that morning, my team of doctors came in to discuss their treatment plan with me and get my consent. There were about six doctors in the room. I'm certain three or four of them were students. I could see the glimmers of excitement in their eyes. "Mr. McKanstry, we have had you on antibiotics, calcium, and fluids. We have found that quite a few patients are showing signs of improvement with an antibody infusion. We would like to take a sample of your blood and match it to the donated antibodies." Antibody infusion. It all sounded strange to me, but I was willing to try it if it helps me get out here and back to my family. "Okay. Let's do it." A few moments later, while the nurse got me set up for my first antibody infusion, Dr. Ritu came in holding a small box in her hand. She gave it to me and said, "When I mentioned that you were looking for a charger, one of the doctors ran out to Best Buy on his lunch break and purchased this for you. He said 'he wanted you to be able to keep in touch with your family.'" You see, this is the kindness that no one would ever know. I never met this doctor to thank him, but his gesture meant the world to me.

As soon as my phone turned on, I video called my family and was thrilled to see my wife and sons. "We miss you, daddy," said Amier.

"Babe, you need to hurry up and come home. These kids are driving me crazy!"

I smiled and laughed because I knew Summer was telling the truth. But honestly, I thought if only I could be home in the midst of the crazy. We made plans to have a family movie night later that evening. By this time, the antibodies were kicking in, which was a strange sensation. I was also getting a lot of other medication through my IV back to back, so I was drained and took a midday nap—something I could never do if I were in the crazy back home.

Later that evening, when I woke up, I decided to check social media, as millions do around the world, and see what was going on. I kept seeing my friends share this post of my former Pastor going live. So I decided to tune in. He played snippets of popular Gospel songs from different church eras, New Mount Zion AME in Tallahassee, FL, where I served as Minister of Music for about four years. Dr. Anton G. Elwood and his wife, Rev. Shawana Elwood, were having a blast. Eventually, they got to the songs that I took part in while serving there, and Pastor Elwood said, "Love you, Jameel." Now, this guy met me when I was a single man, counseled me when I proposed to Summer, married us, and visited and prayed with our first child, and the list goes on and on. He and his wife, Lady Elwood, have been a constant for us.

To be lying in the hospital bed, still on respiratory support, and hearing that I'm loved and appreciated did something for me. It awakened something in me. So I sent him a text to let him know that I appreciated him for everything. In life, I've learned that there's always a reason someone pops into your mind or, as we say in the Christian faith, pops in your spirit. It may be a reminder that a person needs to keep going. So go ahead and send that text or make that phone call to that loved one or friend that randomly pops into your mind. Having lived through a pandemic, you never know what someone is going through. When I texted Pastor Elwood, he told me that he and Lady E were going in prayer immediately. Here he was again, being there for me. What a blessing.

Right after dinner, I was excited to call my wife and check in on her and the boys. "We have the movie all set up." We were getting ready to watch Trolls: World Tour. "How are you feeling, Babe?" my wife asked. "I'm feeling pretty good today. I'm so glad I have a charger. I'm pretty sure one of the nurses was using it earlier today.

Haha!! I bet she's glad I have one too." We laughed, and Summer started the movie. They pointed the phone toward the television so that I could see. This moment was really strange. I was watching a movie with my family on a video call. And even though it felt strange, there was nothing that I'd rather be doing. "Is daddy sleeping?" Amier said. "Yes hun, I think so." I heard just enough of this conversation to remember it, but I was not fully coherent. I'm not sure how long we were on the phone after that, but it mattered to me that my wife stayed on the phone and listened to me snore; that's love.

By Monday, April 27, I had been in the hospital for three days. Today I sat up for a few hours in a chair. I kept hearing Nurse Mary in my head, *Get up. That bed'll hold you.* I walked to the bathroom instead of using the bedside commode. I even washed my face in the sink which was on the far side of the room. I felt like I was getting better. The doctors said they wanted to try me on a smaller breathing tube to see how I would do with that. When the nurse put this on me, I was pleased to no longer have that large mask on my face. But, it took some getting used to.

"Okay, Big Daddy. I'm gonna be taking care of you today. My name is Rashida." Nurse Rashida was a heavy-set woman with short hair and golden skin. She reminded me of some of the women that took care of me growing up, so I believed her when she said she'd be taking care of me. "It's time for your calcium, blood pressure medicine, and I'm going to start the drip for your antibiotics." It sounds like a lot because it was. Every morning this was my routine. And yes, this is after the six-in-the-morning blood samples and the shot in my thigh for the blood thinner. In routine conversation, I decided to ask Nurse Rashida a little bit about her background. Just as I suspected, she was from the South. Tennessee, to be exact. In fact, every nurse that took care of me was from the South. Georgia, Alabama, Mississippi, and Florida. They were my angels. They had to be to come to the epicenter of a global pandemic. They were putting themselves at risk every day to save lives like mine. I have such fond memories of positive exchanges every day with Nurse Rashida. Sometimes I wasn't even in her care, but she made sure to look my way just to make sure I was progressing.

One day, we talked about Greek Letter organizations. As I mentioned, I'm a member of Alpha Phi Alpha Fraternity, Inc., the first black Greek Letter Organization. Nurse Rashida was a Member of Alpha Kappa Alpha Sorority, Inc. (AKA)., the first Black sorority. So naturally, they are recognized as our sister organization. Once I found out she was an AKA, I quickly pulled up their stroll song, "Set It Off," and she started strolling. Here we were in my hospital room, and my nurse was doing her sorority dance. It was an unforgettable moment that brought a lot of joy to my day.

The nurses and PCAs at Elmhurst hospital made me feel special. They took the time to talk with me and encourage me. Someone told me every day that they were going to help get me back home to my wife and kids. I had to jump several hurdles before I could go home. They wanted me to be able to breathe on my own or with a very small amount of oxygen. Every day, I practiced breathing on my own by simply taking off the oxygen and taking those deep breaths Nurse Mary talked about. I had a few key people who checked in with me every day. I did not take this lightly. This is in addition to my wife and sons, who checked in all day every day.

My mom is Shelly McGee. She called every single day. "Hey Mel. How you feeling suga." I'm over thirty years old, and I can't help but smile when my mom calls. Black men and single moms have a special relationship. It's an unspoken bond. A mutual relationship based on the idea of the mom taking care of the kid, but also the kid taking care of the mom. I had to be about six years old on a dark rainy day in Tuscaloosa, AL. I remember my mom and I were coming home from church, and I had a thought and just went with it. "Mom, where's my dad?" "Son, you know your dad, and I don't speak. He was extremely abusive, and I did everything I could to get us away safely." My oldest brother, Ken, who was twenty at the time, was a junior at Southern University, and my middle brother, Dawan, had just left to start his freshman year at the same college as Ken. So growing up, it was mostly mom and me. I responded to her, "I'm so sorry you went through that mom. But don't worry. God is going to send you a good husband." Not soon after, my mom started dating and later married, Bruce McGee, my stepdad who was essential on my life's journey and taken too soon by lung cancer. Throughout our nearly fifteen years together, Mr. Bruce (as I affectionately called him) taught me many valuable lessons. Most of them he never spoke about-he lived them. He was the epitome of a hard-working man who desired so greatly to give his family the best life had to offer. He worked over thirty years at Michelin/BF Goodrich, making tires. Every time I see a set of their tires, I think of him, and the time he took to father me and make sure I had the best of everything. That was emotional. *OK*—Back to the story.

Usually, the next person that would check-in would be my boss, Brian Zager. He's the principal of Lafayette Academy, and he made sure that I knew that he and my colleagues were thinking of me.

My brothers, Dawan and Ken, would check on me every day. Last but certainly not least, one of my best friends from high school, Cleveland "Dee Dee" DuBose, checked on me along with my line brothers.

And the list goes on and on. I'm sharing this with you because as I was going through this sickness alone in this hospital, I would sometimes get overwhelmed by the amount of love and support I received. To every person that reached out to me-THANK YOU. You are a part of why I was encouraged to keep going-THANK YOU. Each night I had a special song that I listened to before I went to sleep and woke up. "I'm Still Here" by Dorinda Clark Cole." In this song, Ms. Dorinda sings about all of the hard times that many people have faced and will continue to face. She ends each verse with "but I'm still here, and it's by the grace of God." I used this song every day to remind myself that it is not of my own doing, but I'm still breathing and still alive because of the grace of God.

As the days went by, my breathing steadily improved. The doctors and nurses were able to steadily decrease my oxygen support, which meant that I was starting to breathe independently. Each time it was decreased, I felt uncomfortable, and I would just check in with the nurse to see if anything was wrong. Finally, nurse Mary said to me, "Of course you're going to feel some discomfort. This will require your lungs to get stronger so they can support you breathing more since they have less support. Just keep taking deep breaths. It'll get easier." Life lesson. Don't panic when things aren't comfortable. Sometimes life will push you to what feels like your limits just to help you stretch and grow. "Just keep taking deep breaths, and it'll get easier." Sure enough, it got easier and more manageable. By May 2, the nurse informed me that they would have me go without oxygen to see how long I could make it. I made it to the early afternoon before I had to call for help. I felt down on myself, but another one of the nurses came to me and said, "We'll try again tomorrow." On May 3, the nurse removed my oxygen tube just after breakfast at around seven-thirty. The doctors came around for their daily checks. "Mr. McKanstry," one doctor said, "You are looking great. Your blood oxidation numbers are looking great. If this stays on track, you'll be able to go home tomorrow." The high nineties are the target for this. This day, my blood oxidation was around ninety-five or ninety-six. Early afternoon came, and I was feeling great. I got up to use the bathroom and stretched from time to time. It was time for dinner, and the sun was starting to set. I was feeling great. I made it all day without oxygen. The doctors confirmed that I would be going home the next day, May 4.

MAY 4, 2021
Elmhurst Hospital
DAY 10

WAS SO EXCITED, AND MY FAMILY WAS ELATED. I CALLED THEM as soon as I got the confirmation that I'd be coming home. "Daddy, I can't wait to see you when you come home. I've missed you so much," exclaimed my oldest, Amier. Caden just looked and smiled. "I'll see you soon, too, Caden." "Babe, I'm so thankful you're coming home. Let me know when you get here," Summer said in an excited tone. We said the I love you's, as we normally do, but this time there was more sincerity and intentionality perhaps than ever before, then we hung up. I took a second and just basked in the silence. If you have kids or have been around kids, you know silence is a blessing. I knew this kind of silence was fleeting so I savored every bit of it I could. I closed my eyes, took deep breaths, and said a simple prayer. "God, I thank you. Thank you for keeping me. Thank you for my family. Bless this day and let it be what you would have it to be in Jesus' name, Amen."

Like most people, our family doesn't usually post challenging times on social media. However, I think it's important to post some bad news because if not, you contribute to the endless scroll of happiness that people see and quietly envy as they think about their own rough times. So I decided to take a picture once I received the details of me going home. I put back on the clothes I came to the hospital in. The gray camouflage pants, my gray Brooklyn hoodie-I have no connection to Brooklyn. I just really like that hoodie. I wrote this post on **FB** that day.

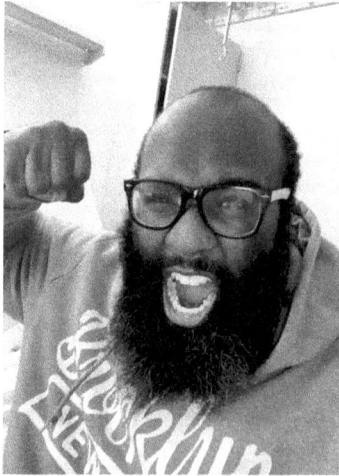

I survived COVID-19. Maybe that doesn't mean anything to you, but it shows me the undeniable power of God. I had been sick for twelve days before I went to the hospital. I had multiple virtual doctor appointments where I got

some prescriptions, but I just was not getting better. On Friday, April 24, I made the tough 911 call because I had some difficulty breathing. Here I thought they'd give me the COVID test, hold me a couple of days, and then I'll be back home. I had no idea how sick I was and how damaged my lungs were. I spent ten days in the hospital. I just started breathing on my own yesterday 5/3. I'm sharing this in hopes that anyone who needs a reason to take this virus seriously takes a look at my story. Black people, men especially, this hits us differently. I have no underlying health issues (high blood pressure, diabetes, asthma), and this virus really took a toll on me. But I thank God I can breathe on my own. And I thank God that I lived to tell the story! Today, I'm headed home.

The only reason that I made it through this was my wife. She FaceTimed me everyday, all day. Sometimes too much. She is taking care of our boys and making sure that they have what they need. Summer McKanstry, I am nothing without you. Thank you for ALWAYS stepping up to the plate and taking care of us! My wife is a SUPERHERO. Wonder Woman ain't got nothing on you babe!

To the nurses, doctors, custodians, social workers, respiratory therapists, specialists. THANK YOU! I did not have one nurse who was from NY. They were all giving of their time from states like Tennessee, Mississippi, Georgia, Florida, and I even had some hometown ladies from Alabama.

They got me right y'all, and made sure I was on the mend.
#frontline #covidsurvivor

I have nearly 5,000 followers on a particular platform. I could get maybe 100 likes and a few comments on a typical day if it were a special post. However, today, I received an outpouring of love and support that I'll never forget. THANK YOU to each person who took time out of their day to pray for me, reach out to help my family, send money, toys, or even just comment a well wish on this post. After many details were ironed out, I was going home. I was instructed to keep taking my blood thinners, sleep on my CPAP, and quarantine for another week.

Like so many people, I watched the news often and would see the reports of how all the nurses would line up in the halls and celebrate the patient leaving. Well, that's not exactly how things went for me. When transportation arrived, I had already packed my belongings. There were two important items I added. The first, was the bright green blanket I was wrapped in when I first arrived at the hospital and told them I was cold. The second was the brand new phone charger one of the doctors (whom I never met) ran out to buy for me; Such a special and touching act of kindness. Both of these items will serve as a reminder of my time here at Elmhurst Hospital and the kindness I was shown. I walked to the stretcher. They double-checked my name and birthdate and strapped me in. Here was my moment.

I wondered how many nurses would be there to send me off. As we turned the corner to go toward the elevator, I saw one lonely nurse who asked, "Are you going home?" I was shocked! Really?? THIS WAS IT?? All I could do was laugh and confirm that I was indeed going home. "Wait one second." She ran and grabbed one other staff member, and they clapped for me and played a cowbell. It was really sad, but I played along, smiled, and celebrated. I think even one of the transport guys was laughing. Once the elevator door closed, I burst into laughter. I couldn't help it.

Then, I came to my senses and thought. *I wonder how many people went into this hospital, but never came out.* Gratefulness hit me like a ton of bricks as I was wheeled through the lobby of the hospital. On our way out, several people greeted and congratulated me for being on the other side of COVID-19. The automatic doors opened. We were outside. Now what's interesting is this whole time I knew I was at Elmhurst Hospital. I just had no idea where Elmhurst hospital was until this moment. *Oh,* I thought to myself. *This is where I am.* As I was being wheeled to the ambulance, I saw some familiar fast-food restaurants and the 7-train where I dropped off Summer a number of times. This was a beautiful day. There was a slight chill in the air. It felt good to breathe some fresh air. I was going home. I beat COVID. Everything was getting back to normal.

The ambulance pulled in front of our home and dropped me off. I made sure to have all of my belongings-I definitely could not chase this ambulance down the street. Almost as soon as I was on my feet, the ambulance was gone. Here I was. Alone. One thing about the homes in New York is that they have a lot of stairs. When I lived down South, stairs meant wealth and luxury so common people, didn't really have stairs in their homes. Outside there are ten steps. On a normal day, I don't even think about walking up the steps. I just do it. But today, I had to take my time and climb each one. ONE… TWO…EIGHT…NINE…TEN. That was just to get to the front door. I had to take a break before I continued climbing the fifteen stairs that waited inside for me. These accurate numbers were provided by my Ma, who knows all too well how many steps it takes to get inside our apartment. You see, we live in what's called a multi-family home where although there is only one physical building, there are a few different apartments within the home. So to get inside, there are a total of twenty-five stairs to climb. Finally, I built up enough strength to continue the long haul upstairs. By the time I got to the top of the stairs, I was winded again. "YOU'RE HERE!!! I wasn't expecting you so soon!" I was met with the smiling eyes of Summer and our two boys. They were so happy to see me, and the feeling was beyond mutual. I was happy to be home, back in the crazy. We both had masks, and Summer met me holding a garbage bag for my clothes. I had to immediately get undressed and take a shower. You need to wash that hospital off of you, exclaimed Summer. While in the hospital, I asked the nurses every day to help wipe me down and change my sheets. **PRO-TIP:** When you (or a loved one) are in the hospital, ask the nurses to wash you and change your sheets daily. Also, if you can, sit in a chair for some hours each day. This helps prevent bedsores which are no fun. I lathered up my body with my favorite soap. It smells fresh and feels great. As I was rinsing off the first time-yes, I did multiple washes. I noticed the brown liquid quickly rushing down the drain. *Damn I'm dirty.* I thought to myself and proceeded to wash a couple more times. I was feeling tired and drained, so I thought I'd better hurry. I was lifting my foot when I lost my balance. In a panic, I quickly grabbed onto the wall and could barely save myself from a nasty fall. I was embarrassed. I pulled myself together, dried off, and decided to weigh myself. Before COVID, I was 386 pounds. After being sick for about three weeks and hospitalized for ten days, I was 346 pounds. Losing weight when you're sick can be so scary and can make you feel like everything is out of your control. On my way to my quarantine chambers, I saw my Mother-In-Law or, Ma. We chatted briefly about how I was doing and that she prayed for me and was so glad that I was on the mend. I headed upstairs-YEP more stairs to get to my bedroom.

As I walked into the room, tears started to roll down my face. My wife had cleaned and disinfected the room from top to bottom. The room was spotless. This is not how it was left. From bodily waste to all sorts of germs, I could write all day about how grateful I am for the amount of preparation

Summer made for me. The last time I was in this room, I was sick and nearly out of my mind. But here I was, back at home and feeling much better. We have a King size bed. I mean-I'm a big guy. I grabbed my huge pillow that allows me to sit upright and put it on the bed. We have a small refrigerator upstairs that Summer stocked with water, juice, and ginger ale.

I grabbed some water and sat down to watch some internet-streamed TV. I saw The Blacklist, a show I stopped watching quite a few seasons back. I decided I'd use these days to catch up. The storylines are so crazy that each character has their own secrets. The murders are hardly ever the same. I just love how Megan Boone portrays Elizabeth Keen, the daughter of a Russian spy, who is now a part of a special task force that has partnered with a man who claims to be Raymond Reddington. Raymond Reddington is the most wanted criminal in the world for the countless crimes that he committed. There is something about this brilliant play on good and evil, and the gray area in between that intrigues me and keeps me coming back for more.

My phone rings. "Babe, you hungry? I'm cooking some food." In what seemed like a few minutes, I heard a knock on the door. "Honey, your food is out here. Love you!" I did my best to call out and say, "Thank you!" Even though I could breathe on my own, I still became winded very easily. So I got up from the bed and went to get my food. What was normally a task that took ten seconds and hardly any thought had become a task that had to be planned for and thought about. I opened the door, picked up the food, and took my time getting back to the bed. I do not remember exactly what Summer cooked, but I know it was some of my favorite foods. It was too much food. I ate a little and reminded my love "Hey babe, I know I usually eat big plates of food, I can't even handle half of this. But that's okay. I can eat some more of it later. The food was so good." I was happy to be home, but I had second thoughts about my breathing. Certain things just weren't feeling right. For instance, when I tried to lay down and go to sleep, I couldn't breathe as well. Even with my CPAP, a machine prescribed for sleep apnea, I still felt uncomfortable, like I couldn't quite catch my breath. So I adjusted. I grabbed my giant upright pillow and sat up to go to sleep. It definitely took some getting used to, but I eventually dozed off watching an episode of The Blacklist.

For nearly two weeks, my wife cooked every meal for us: breakfast, lunch, and dinner. She waited on me, hand and foot. If I needed more water or some hot tea, she took care of it. When I felt alone, she would sit on a video call with me. Sometimes I didn't want to talk, and I just wanted to be in the presence of another human. She kept me grounded during this most difficult time.

Usually, I talk to my mom every day. This was especially true while I was in the hospital, and it remained when I came back home. My mom even learned how to video chat. She was so happy to be able to see me. "You're looking good son, but you need to shave." I tell you, there is no shade like good ol' Southern shade. They slide you a compliment just to tell you something that's not quite right. All I could do was laugh. Truthfully, I was (am) still traumatized by trying to shave in high school, destroying my beard, and starting over. From that day to this one, I leave it to the professionals. "Okay Momma, I have to quarantine first, but I'll take care of it." In a quiet, sweet tone, she told me, "Son, I am so thankful to God for keeping you safe during this virus. I prayed for you every day. That God would bless you and keep you. That He would always surround you with the right people that mean you well. And that's just what He did in that hospital. Thank you Lord." I'm pretty sure she started singing a song. I tried to laugh it off, but the truth is I was touched by what she said. After all these years, to know that my Mother is still praying for me. This doesn't get old. I'm forever grateful for moments like this.

On May 14, I was able to come around the family, but all the women in my life agreed that I should keep on my mask for a few more days just in case. Today was the first day I had a hug in over a month. I hugged my wife, hugged Amier, and held little Caden. It was beautiful. I was beyond thankful to be back home, back to the crazy. Honestly, there was no place I'd rather be. One day, I hope everyone who touched my life during this scary time can read these words. So I'm going to close with some words of thanks.

God,

Thank You for life. You are the source of all things. Everything comes from you. I am nothing without you. Thank you for every talent and gift you have placed in me. I will use it for your glory and the good of all humanity.

Summer,

Thank you for loving me. You have always held a special place in my heart. I love you today and every day. You are beautiful, kind, talented, and fierce. You are perfect in every way. Stay strong throughout the hard times. They don't last. But our love will last forever.

Amier,

You have always been a ball of energy. Keep the energy, but harness it for good. You have great power, great influence; use it wisely. You are beautiful. You are bold. You are brave. There's nothing you can't do. Take care of yourself. Take care of your family. Always remember your faith. I love you.

Caden,

What a beam of light and goodness you are. You have the power to shift a room when you walk in. Never seek validation from anyone. Validate yourself. You are enough. Find your passion and go after it with everything in you. I love you.

Mom (Shelly),
You brought me into this world. We have been through so much together, and we're still going strong. You inspire me. I love you.

Brothers (Ken and Dawan),
You two inspire me and teach me. Thanks for always being there for my family and me. I love you both.

Ma (Roberta),
Thank you for picking up the slack and filling in the gaps. I could never thank you enough for all you have been to our family. I love you.

Justice and Jaclyn Hall,
Thank you for checking on me and helping us out. You both are always there when we need you, which goes beyond words. You two inspire me, and I'm so thankful to be a part of your life. Love ya'll.

Pastor Elwood and New Mount Zion AME-Tallahassee,
Thank you for being a constant in my life. You have always pushed me to be the absolute best I can be, whether I think I can or not. I am forever indebted to you.

Mike Bailey (#7), Front,
Thank you for checking in with me often. You've been a constant since 2007. I love you Bro, and I'm so proud of you.

Chris Forde (#9), Back,
You already know what it is. Thank you for the love and support. I'm blessed to call you Brother.

Cleveland "DeeDee" DuBose,
Thank you, Brother for your kindness to my family and me. So grateful to have you in my life.

Amanda Chin and Friends at Afterwork Theater,
Thank you for your love and support.

Pastor Gardner and East Ward,
Thank you for your prayers and continued support.

To you,
Thank you for reading this book. I hope that you have some bits of information you can use on your journey. Be kind to yourself and be kind to others. Love yourself. Love others. Believe in God (if you choose) but always believe in yourself (that's not an option).

With Love,
Jameel A. McKanstry

Author Bio

JAMEEL McKANSTRY IS A SINGER/SONGWRITER, TEACHER, and author. Hailing from Tuscaloosa, AL, McKanstry earned his Bachelor's of Music Education Degree specializing in Choral Music from Florida State University. McKanstry relocated to New York City and earned his Master's Degree in Educational Theatre at New York University. McKanstry teaches in the New York City public school system and is the Songwriting Lead for Music Unlimited Entertainment, LLC, a full-service music publishing company.

www.ingramcontent.com/pod-product-compliance
Lightning Source LLC
Chambersburg PA
CBHW060258030426
42335CB00014B/1767